Smile!

Your Guide to Esthetic Dental Treatment

Douglas A. Terry, DDS

Editorial Assistant
Melissa Nix

Advisors
John O. Burgess, DDS, MS
Susana B. Paoloski, DDS
Rocio Barocio, DDS
Kim S. Gee, DDS, MS
Alejandro James, DDS, MSD
Mark L. Stankewitz, DDS, CDT
Victor Castro, CDT

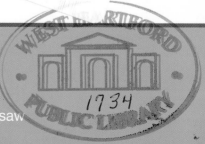

quintessence
books

Quintessence Publishing Co, Inc

Chicago, Berlin, Tokyo, London, Paris, Milan, Barcelona, Beijing,
Istanbul, Moscow, New Delhi, Prague, São Paulo, Seoul, Singapore, and Warsaw

I would like to express my gratitude to my dedicated team—Melissa Nix, Ernesto de Haro Tostado, and Rocio Barocio—for their relentless work ethic and continued commitment to excellence. A great deal of thanks to my family of patients who continue to actively participate in decisions regarding their dental care and to ask important questions for their improved oral health and proper decision making, without whom this book would not be possible. This project would not have seen daylight without the dedication, organization, and imagination of Captain Leah Huffman, Sue Robinson, Ted Pereda, Angelina Sanchez, Lisa Bywaters, and Kristina Hartman from the Quintessence team. Also, a special recognition to Sue Terry, who is not only my mother but also my best friend and my most attentive critic. Most important, to my Creator who makes me realize that teeth and gums are simple in His hands but so complex in mine.

Library of Congress Cataloging-in-Publication Data
Terry, Douglas A., author.
Smile! : your guide to esthetic dental treatment / Douglas A. Terry.
   p. ; cm.
Your guide to esthetic dental treatment
ISBN 978-0-86715-667-6
I. Title. II. Title: Your guide to esthetic dental treatment.
[DNLM: 1. Esthetics, Dental--Popular Works. WU 80]
RK60.7
617.6'01--dc23
                          2013049340

quintessence
books

© 2014 Quintessence Publishing Co Inc

Quintessence Publishing Co Inc
4350 Chandler Drive
Hanover Park, IL 60133
www.quintpub.com

5 4 3 2 1

Editor: Leah Huffman
Design: Ted Pereda
Production: Angelina Sanchez

A special thank you to the clinical and laboratory contributors:

Willi Geller, MDT

Olivier Tric, MDT

Juan José Gutierréz Riera, DDS, MSD

Alex H. Schuerger, CDT

Tetsuji Aoshimo, DDS

Francisco Zárate, DDS, CDT

August Bruguera, CDT

Charles Moreno, MDT, CDT

Jungo Endo, RDT

Richard Young, DDS

Michael K. McGuire, DDS

Upgrading your smile begins with good oral health. Healthy gums and a well-aligned bite underlie any beautiful smile. Enhancing your smile can be as easy as a simple bleaching procedure to improve tooth color or an uncomplicated bonding technique to change tooth shape. More invasive approaches may involve surgery to change gum line contours, tooth alignment with braces, or replacement of missing teeth with partial dentures, implants, or complete dentures. There are a variety of restoration methods to ensure a healthy smile: composite bonding, veneers, inlays, onlays, and crowns. Tooth-colored composite resin and ceramics are materials often used to restore teeth to a natural, attractive look. Selection of the most appropriate materials depends on the amount of tooth structure being replaced.

You may have one or more of the following questions about your smile and oral health:

- Are my front teeth too short for my smile?
- How can excessive gaps between my front teeth be reduced?
- What options do I have to align my crowded teeth?
- Can bleaching improve my stained teeth? Should it be performed before any other treatment?
- What foods and drinks will stain my teeth and new restorations?
- How do I prevent and manage tooth sensitivity?
- What are the options for fixing my fractured front tooth?
- Do missing teeth affect my bite?
- Is there a way to change my "gummy smile"?
- How can my unattractive gum line be corrected?
- Can my denture appear more natural and fit better when I chew?
- Will correcting my bite and smile improve my health, appearance, and self-confidence?

The purpose of this book is to answer questions like these and to illustrate different available treatment options. Your smile is composed of all of the teeth and gums that are exposed when you speak or smile broadly. I hope the illustrations in this book help you to make decisions about restoring and maintaining a healthy and pleasing smile.

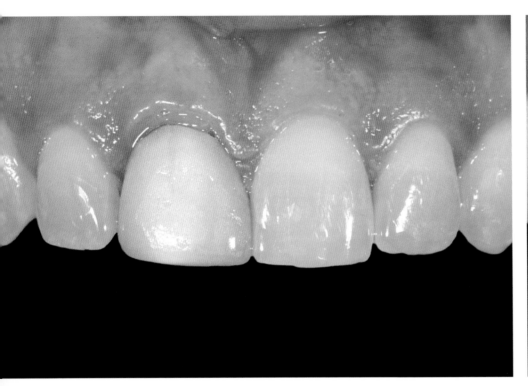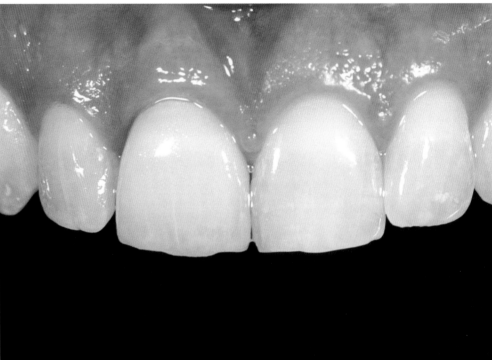

An attractive smile displays the upper front teeth, so if an esthetic smile is the goal, the shape, length, color, and contour of these teeth are important when restoring your smile. There are several ceramic materials that can be used to fabricate crowns for restoring your front teeth. These include metal-ceramic and all-ceramic crowns. The appropriate material is determined by the color of the underlying tooth and the surrounding teeth. A metal-ceramic or opaque all-ceramic crown such as zirconia can be used to hide discolorations, while a translucent all-ceramic crown can be selected to match the natural color of the underlying tooth color.

This 35-year-old patient was displeased with the dark gray color at the gum line of her front tooth, an existing metal-ceramic crown. The metal substructure of the existing crown was noticeable upon smiling and speaking. An all-ceramic translucent crown was selected for replacement. The patient was pleased with the natural color at the gum line and the improved balance in shape and color of her front teeth.

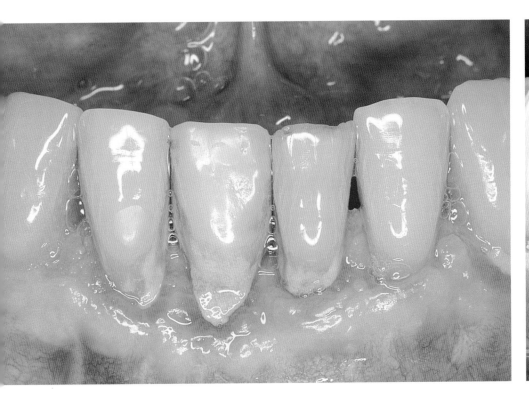 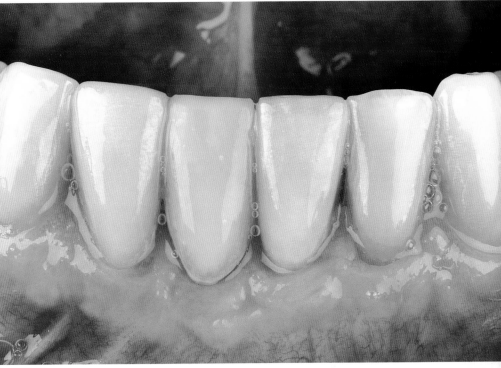

Gum recession is a common concern in adults over the age of 40 years. You may not notice this gradual change because it can be minimal from one day to another. There are many possible causes for gum recession, including periodontal disease, abnormal tooth position due to crowding, overaggressive brushing, improper flossing, thin and fragile gums, eating disorders such as bulimia, dipping tobacco, tongue and lip piercing, and clenching and grinding of your teeth. If not treated, gum recession can eventually cause tooth loss.

There are different types of gum grafts to treat recession, the most common of which is the connective tissue graft. This procedure involves taking tissue from the roof of your mouth and stitching it to the gum tissue around exposed roots. Graft material from a tissue bank can also be used.

This 50-year-old patient had tooth abrasion and gum line recession from overaggressive brushing. His gums and teeth were restored with a gum graft and porcelain veneers, and he was taught improved brushing and flossing techniques with a soft toothbrush and a less abrasive toothpaste.

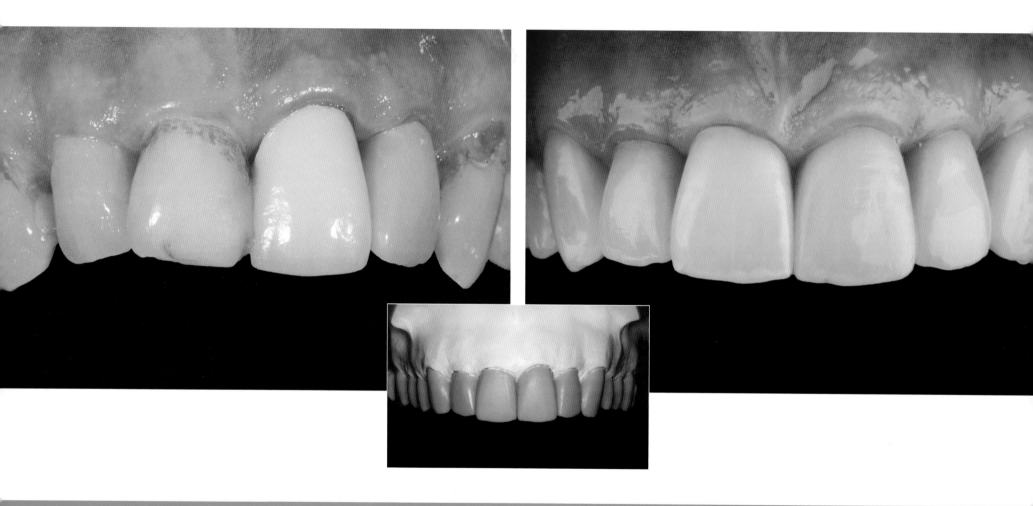

This 52-year-old patient had large, defective tooth-colored fillings on his front teeth and a metal post underlying the existing metal-ceramic crown. He was unhappy with the existing tooth-colored restorations and the mismatch of the crown to his surrounding teeth. A diagnostic wax-up (a wax copy of the anticipated final restored teeth) was designed and served as a prototype for visualization by the patient and fabrication of the definitive restorations. Metal-free, all-ceramic zirconium crowns were selected to restore the front teeth and mask the color of the post.

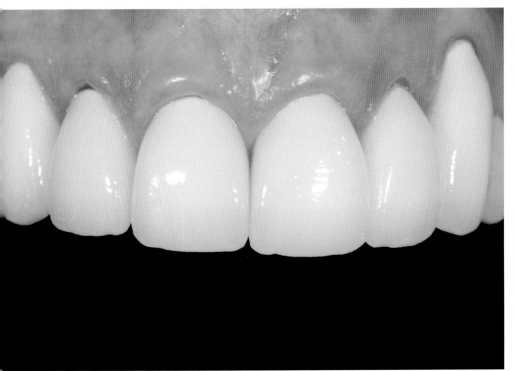 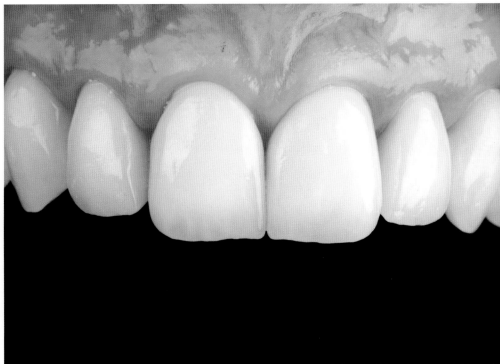

This 60-year-old patient was unhappy with her smile and the extreme prolonged sensitivity after the initial restoration of her teeth by a cosmetic dentist who failed to follow proper restorative guidelines. After cosmetic gum grafting surgery, her teeth were restored with all-ceramic crowns for a more natural and healthy appearance.

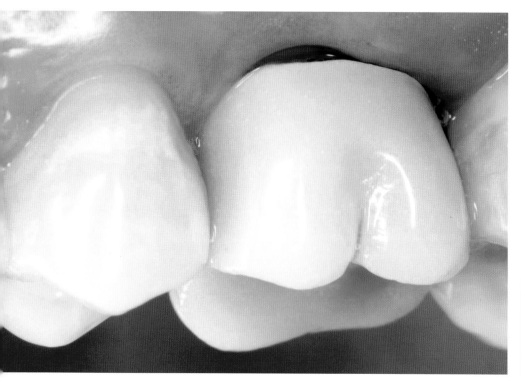
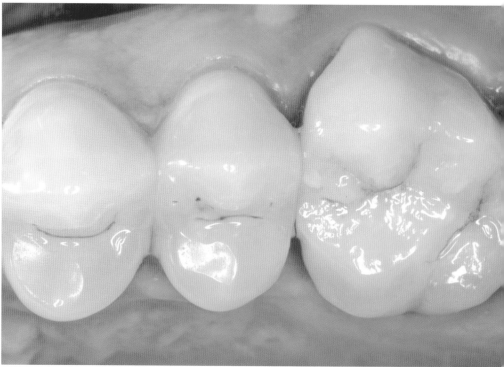

Color discrepancy between the root and the ceramic crown can be noticeable at the gum line. Proper selection and integration of ceramic materials can improve the appearance.

This 45-year-old patient had concerns about the discolored region above her existing ceramic crown, which was noticeable at the gum line when she spoke or smiled. The patient indicated that this was all she saw when she looked in the mirror. The crown was removed, and the existing preparation was modified at the gum line. With such a minor change, this woman was able to share her smile with the world and look into the mirror again with confidence.

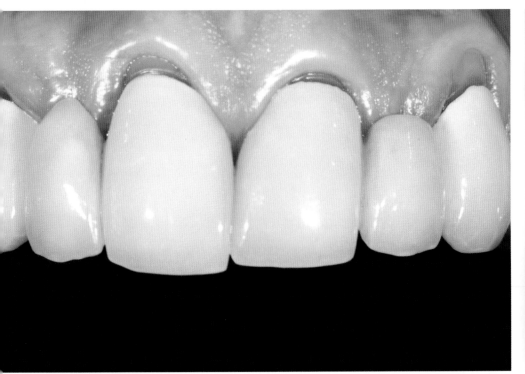 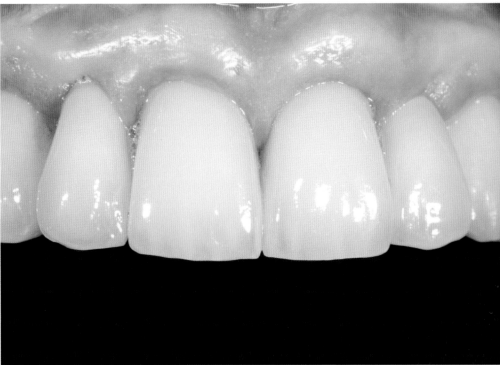

This patient had two three-unit bridges replacing her missing front teeth. The artificial teeth (called *pontics*) appeared unnatural as they emerged from the gums. Gum grafting procedures provided improvement to the gum volume and contour at the necks of her natural teeth and to the pontics of her new metal-ceramic bridges. This dramatic change encouraged her to inspire others to achieve a healthy and beautiful smile.

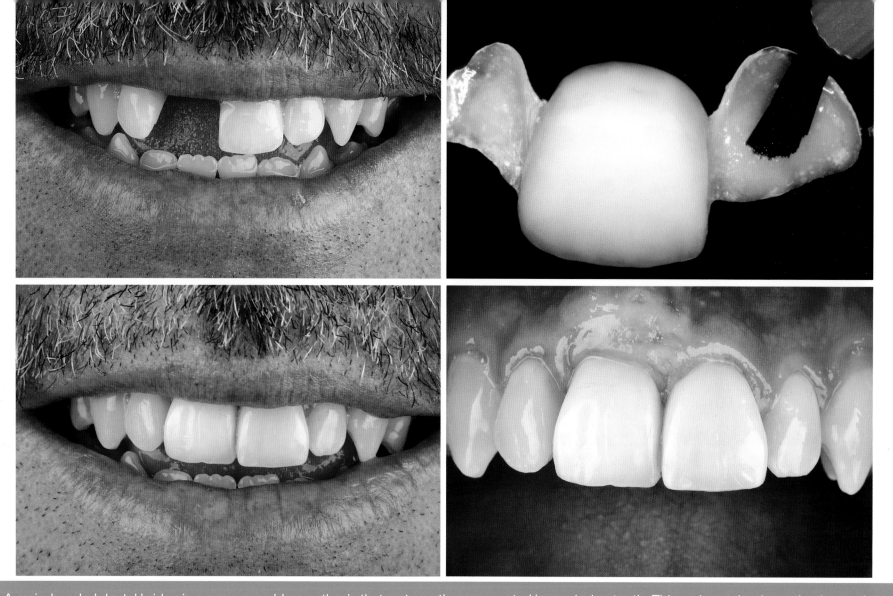

A resin-bonded dental bridge is a nonremovable prosthesis that restores the gap created by a missing tooth. This resin-retained prosthesis consists of a composite-reinforced framework that has wings or retainers that bond to the teeth on either side of the gap (abutment teeth). This treatment concept is increasingly being used as an alternative to more invasive procedures because it replaces missing teeth and restores function and esthetics while requiring minimal preparation. Also, the resin-bonded bridge can be used as a transitional restoration for patients whose age or finances preclude them from implant or conventional bridge placement. In addition, this prosthesis can be used to develop and preserve gum contours (following gum and bone grafting) before implant placement.

This patient lost his front tooth in a sporting accident. The resin-bonded bridge was selected to restore the esthetics and function while the bone and gums were restored to an ideal contour and position with a grafting procedure. After healing, a single-tooth implant was placed, and an implant-supported abutment and crown were fabricated and placed to restore the space and the patient's beautiful smile.

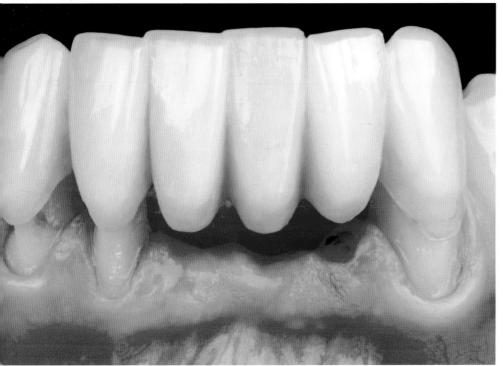
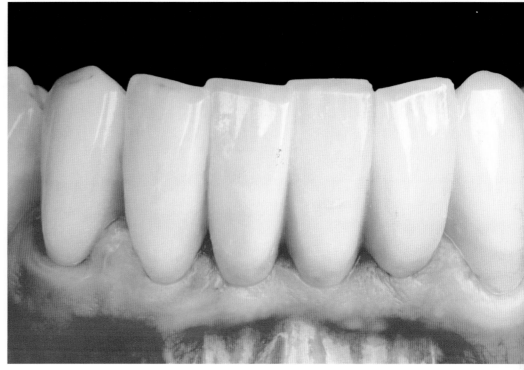

A fixed dental bridge is a nonremovable prosthesis that fills the gap created by one or more missing teeth. A bridge is composed of abutment teeth and pontics. *Abutment teeth* are crowns on teeth or implants on either side of the gap that provide support. *Pontics* are artificial teeth that are shaped and layered from ceramic material onto an underlying framework that is made of gold, alloy, or high-strength ceramic material such as zirconium. Bridges can restore your ability to chew, speak, and smile while distributing uneven forces in your bite and preventing remaining teeth from drifting into the gap.

This patient selected a fixed all-ceramic zirconium bridge to replace her missing lower front teeth. The patient was confident with the function she gained and pleased with the natural appearance.

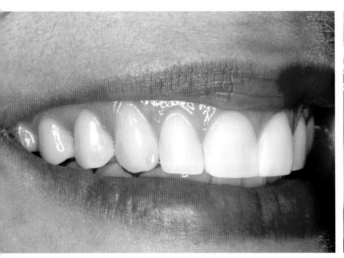 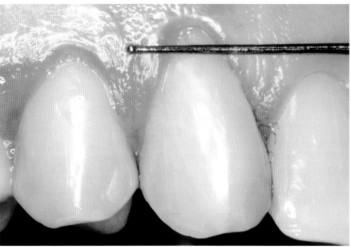 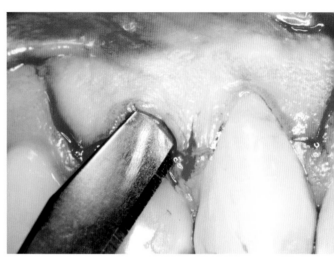

This 35-year-old patient was concerned about the gum recession around her canine. Measurements were taken of the anticipated volume of gum tissue that was needed to cover this recession. An incision was made around the tooth, and the gum tissue was reflected (lifted up).

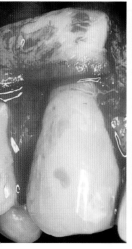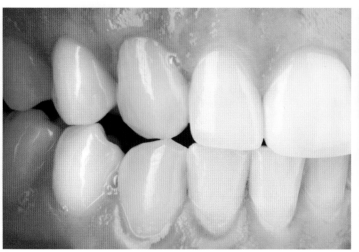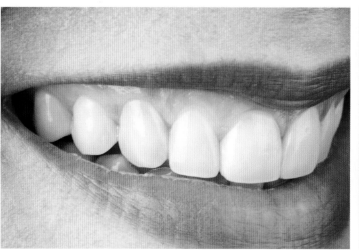

A gum graft of the measured volume taken from the roof of the mouth was then sutured into place around the neck of the tooth, and the lifted gum tissue was repositioned over the graft and sutured. This simple alteration restored this woman's attractive smile.

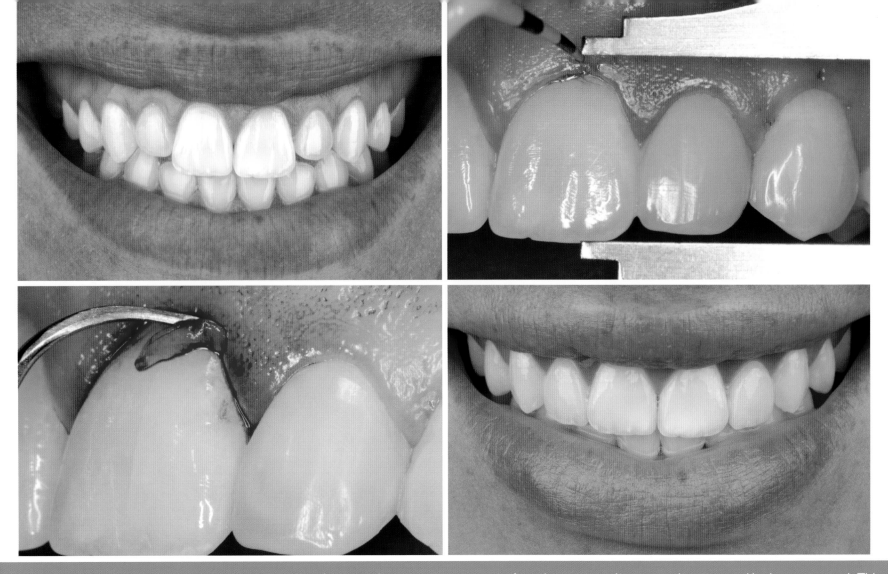

Crown lengthening is a cosmetic surgical procedure for exposing a greater amount of tooth structure. It can require gum and/or bone removal. This procedure may need to be performed after tooth fracture or excessive gum line decay to provide an adequate amount of tooth structure to support a crown. It is used to establish a healthy gum-bone relationship around existing restorations or before replacement. Also, this procedure is used to cosmetically treat a "gummy smile." A *gummy smile* is when an unusual amount of gum tissue shows around the upper teeth when smiling.

This 26-year-old patient was dissatisfied with the size of her lateral incisors and the excess amount of gum tissue that showed when she smiled. Cosmetic gum surgery and two porcelain veneers transformed her smile and raised her self-confidence.

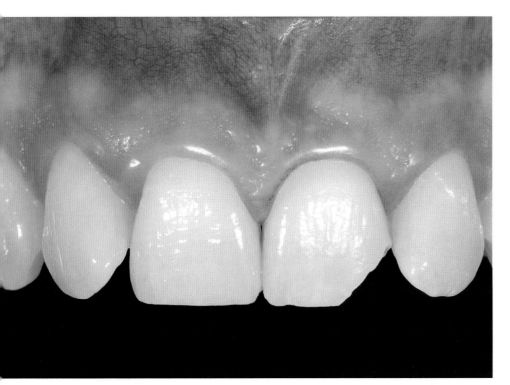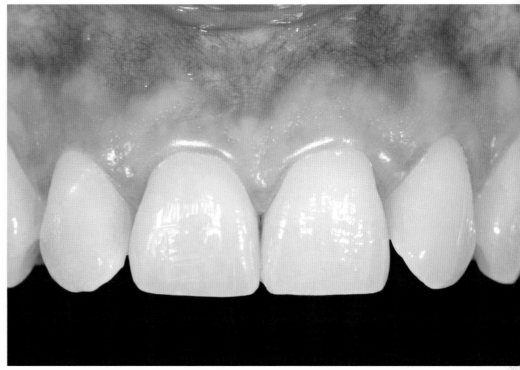

Natural tooth is remarkably strong, but it can chip, fracture, or break from trauma, malposition, biting on unusually hard objects, clenching or grinding, untreated decay, and root canal treatment. Minor tooth fractures may not elicit pain, but extreme discomfort can result from more extensive fractures or displacement. With extensive fractures, the nerve ending may be damaged and/or exposed and may require immediate assessment by your dentist. If the tooth has sharp or jagged edges, cover it with a piece of wax paraffin or sugarless chewing gum to prevent it from cutting your tongue or the inside of your lip or cheek.

Displaced or dislodged teeth should be evaluated immediately by your dentist (within a few hours) for possible replacement or repositioning in the socket and stabilization by splinting. A cold compress should be applied to the injured area, and the tooth should be rinsed with saliva, saline, or milk and placed in the same solution or, if possible, placed in the mouth between the cheek and the jaw or under the tongue.

This 28-year-old patient fractured her front tooth on a peach seed. The tooth was restored with minimal tooth removal and a tooth-colored composite material in one visit. Management of any dental injury after initial treatment requires reevaluation and follow-up to detect changes and complications that can occur.

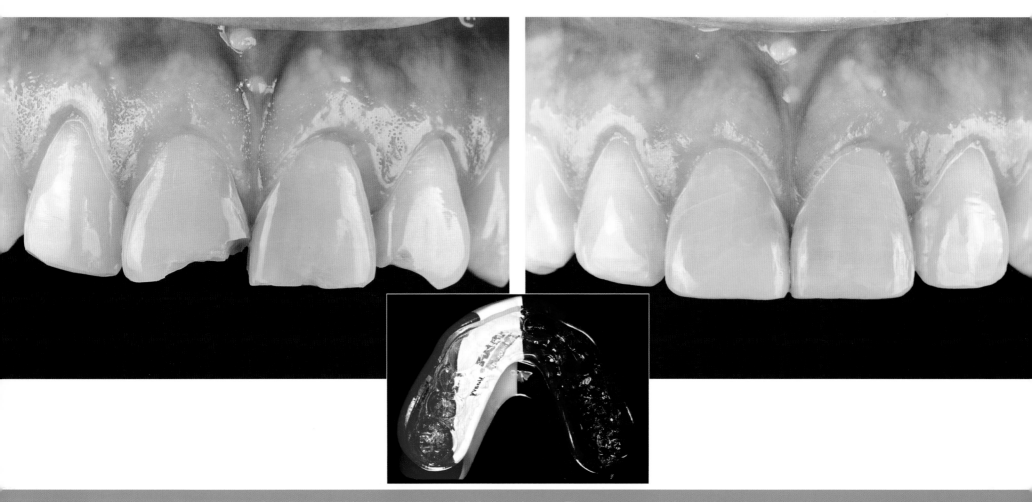

This 26-year-old college student fractured his front teeth in a fall during skating. There was sensitivity to air and cold but no immediate signs of nerve damage upon evaluation and review of the x-ray. The fractured teeth were restored with a tooth-colored composite material, and the patient was given an athletic guard to wear during sporting activities. At 6-week, 3-month, and 18-month follow-up visits, reevaluation indicated no changes or complications, and the patient had no further sensitivity or nerve damage.

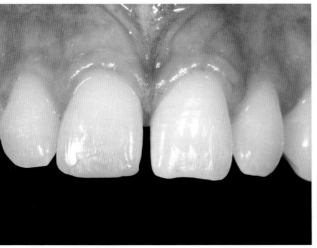
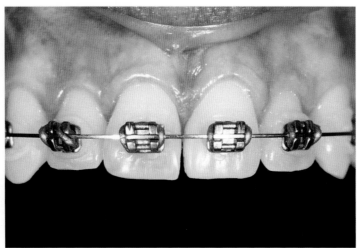
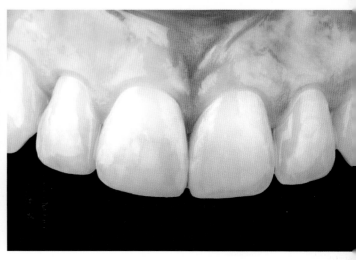

A gap between the teeth is referred to as a *diastema*, and it appears most often between the upper front teeth. These gaps can be caused by a mismatch between the size of the jawbones and the size of the teeth, oversized muscle (frenum) attachments, habits such as thumb sucking, an incorrect swallowing reflex, and periodontal disease. Before treatment, your dentist should determine the reason for the space. Sometimes these gaps are unpleasant to the patient and can be closed with braces and/or dental restorations.

This 39-year-old patient wore braces to close the spaces and selected tooth-colored composite to alter minor esthetic contours of her front teeth.

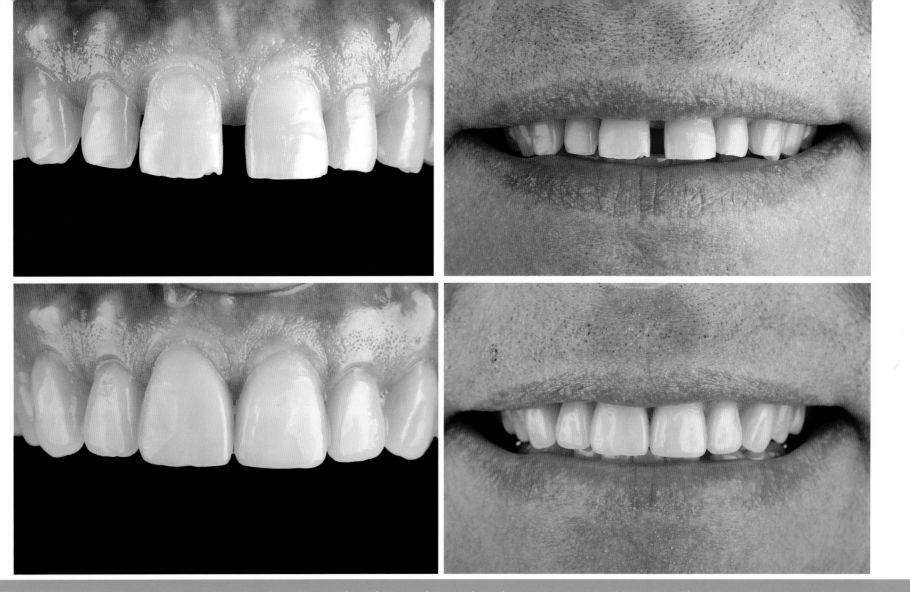

Direct composite bonding is a noninvasive dental procedure that can be used to close gaps, repair chipped and/or decayed teeth, and alter and improve tooth size, shape, length, alignment, color, and contour. Direct bonding is a popular treatment procedure because it requires minimal to no tooth removal and provides a successful and strong attachment between the composite filling material and the tooth enamel and dentin. Direct bonding involves direct application of a tooth-colored composite material to the tooth surface to achieve a desired final shape and color.

This 63-year-old man selected a conservative direct bonding procedure to restore his upper front teeth. The procedure was completed without anesthesia in two dental visits, and the patient was extremely happy with his new younger-looking and attractive smile.

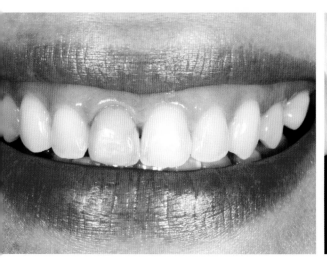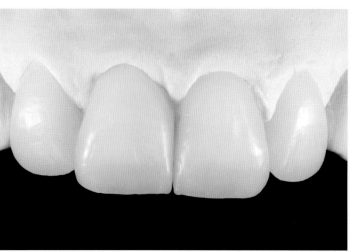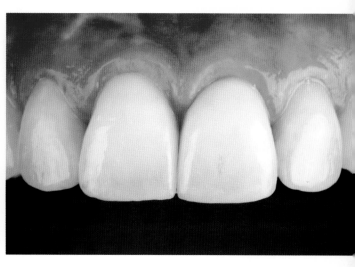

This 44-year-old patient was dissatisfied with her discolored front teeth. The existing tooth-colored fillings were decayed and discolored, and the right central incisor was darker than the surrounding teeth. A tooth that appears darker may indicate that the nerve is injured or dead. The tooth was tested for vitality, and the measurements indicated that it was nonvital (the nerve was dead). A root canal was performed on the tooth to restore health. To balance and disguise the underlying tooth colors of the central incisors and to reinforce the remaining tooth structure, metal-ceramic crowns were placed on the central incisors, and porcelain veneers were placed on the adjacent incisors.

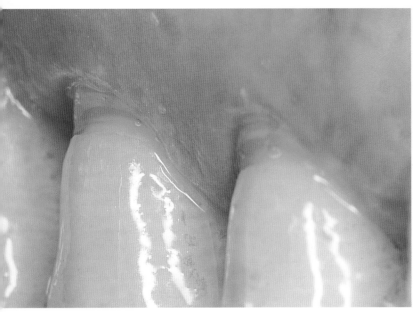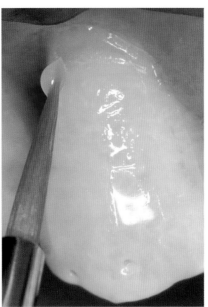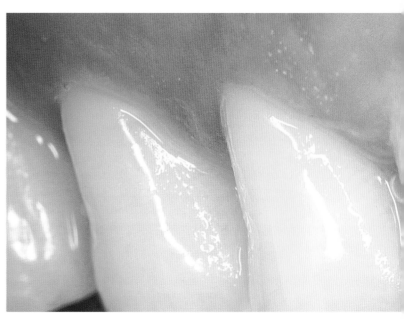

Small notches like these at the gum line can be extremely sensitive to cold temperatures and to tooth brushing. This 46-year-old woman indicated that she drank fruit juices during the day and brushed her teeth rigorously after consumption. A tooth-colored filling called *composite* was bonded to the abraded surface, and the pain was eliminated. The patient was instructed to reduce her acidic beverage consumption and to rinse with water after consuming acidic foods or drinks. She was also instructed not to brush for at least an hour after consumption of any acidic beverage (eg, juice, fruit, soda, coffee, wine).

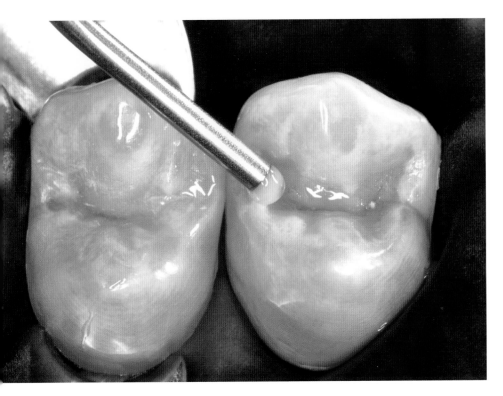
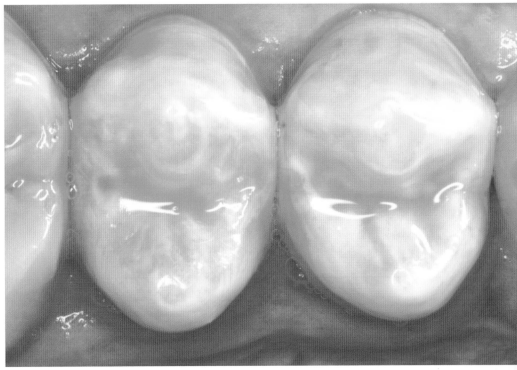

Your back teeth have small grooves called *pits* and *fissures* on their biting surfaces that can become traps for foods and liquids that contain sugar. The sugar can be converted into acid by resident bacteria in plaque and demineralize the tooth surface, causing a cavity. Dental sealants are thin, plastic coatings that can be applied to these grooves. This coating protects the chewing surfaces from tooth decay by keeping bacteria and food particles out of the grooves.

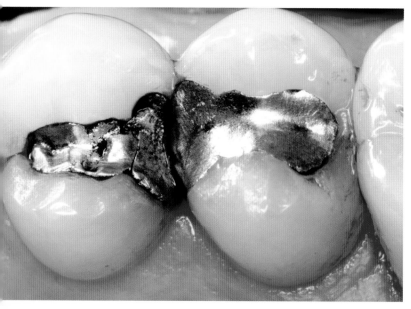 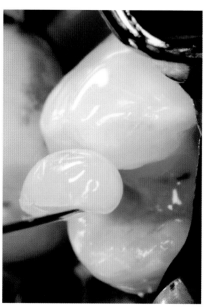 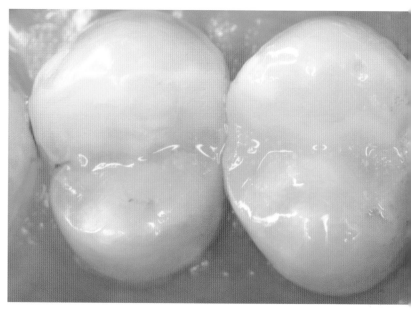

Dental amalgam fillings, also known as *silver fillings* because of their silverlike appearance, have been used for more than 150 years to fill cavities. However, the silver appearance can distract from a beautiful smile. Composite resin is the most common alternative restorative material for the replacement of dental amalgam and requires minimal removal of healthy tooth structure for placement. The color of composite can be customized to closely match your surrounding teeth.

This 60-year-old woman was concerned about the noticeable gray discoloration between her teeth when talking and smiling. She selected a tooth-colored direct composite filling as a conservative and esthetic choice that required a treatment time of only 2 hours.

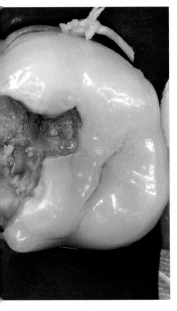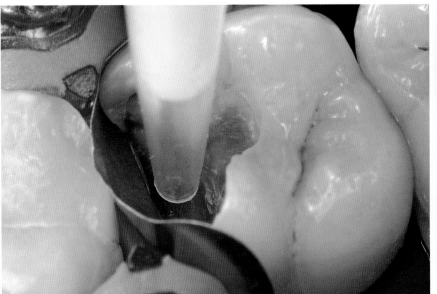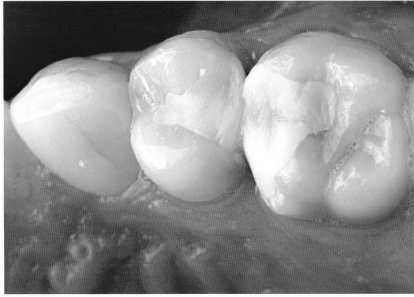

The primary reason for tooth structure replacement on existing restorations is recurring tooth decay. Aggressive forms of tooth decay are usually associated with inadequate salivary output or frequent exposure to fermentable carbohydrates. To reduce the potential of tooth decay, bioactive filling materials can be placed into the cavity to serve as a reservoir for fluoride.

Because of this patient's high decay rate, a resin-modified glass ionomer (a bioactive, fluoride-releasing intermediate material) was selected to reduce decay. This material is similar to composite resin, but its fluoride-releasing therapeutic effect aids in the management of tooth decay on the affected and adjacent teeth.

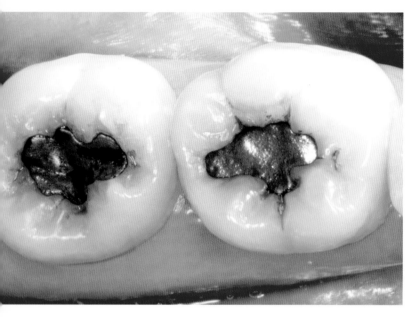
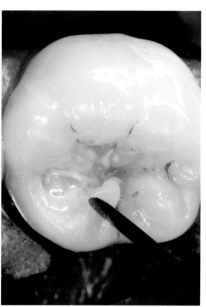
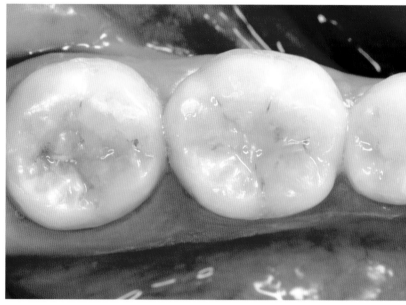

These amalgam fillings lasted 20 years, but the seal between the filling and the tooth opened, leading to decay and therefore requiring replacement. The main advantages of a direct tooth-colored composite filling over metallic materials such as amalgam are minimal tooth structure removal and improved esthetics. Composites come in a variety of tooth colors, allowing for an indistinguishable result. These materials are bonded into the tooth, which strengthens the tooth structure. It is important to know that composite fillings wear from chewing, grinding, and clenching and can require resurfacing or replacement. Your dentist should routinely check your existing fillings for surface wear.

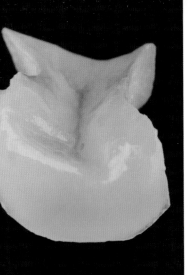

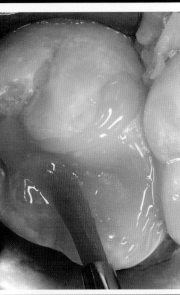

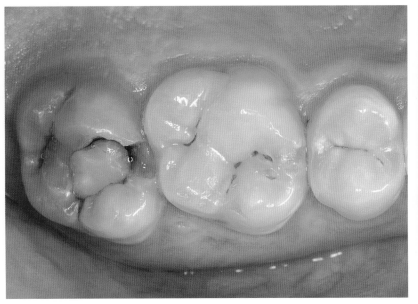

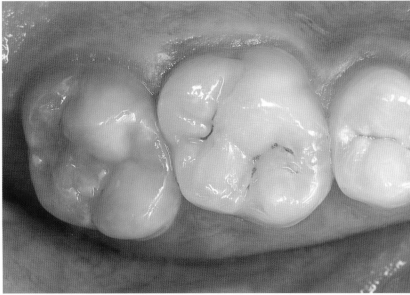

Inlays are custom-made internal fillings that are fabricated in the laboratory from a conventional or digital impression of the prepared cavity in the mouth. These cavity inserts can be made of composite, porcelain, or gold. The advantages of these indirect restorations are superior fit, improved contours, and increased durability. These inserts are usually selected to replace and repair moderate tooth decay or recurring decay on existing cracked or worn fillings. The insert is bonded inside the cavity with adhesive cement, which can strengthen the damaged or weakened areas of the tooth. These restorations are usually prepared and fabricated in two visits to the dentist, but some dentists have computer-aided design and manufacturing systems that allow fabrication and cementation in one visit.

This patient had only one moderately decayed region on the upper second molar that extended into the flossing area of the molars. A composite inlay was selected to provide controlled contours for ideal flossing in this area.

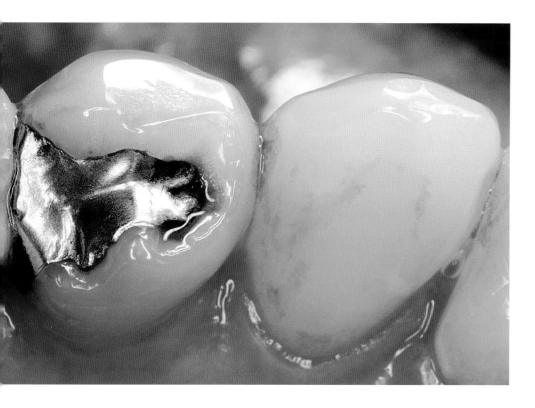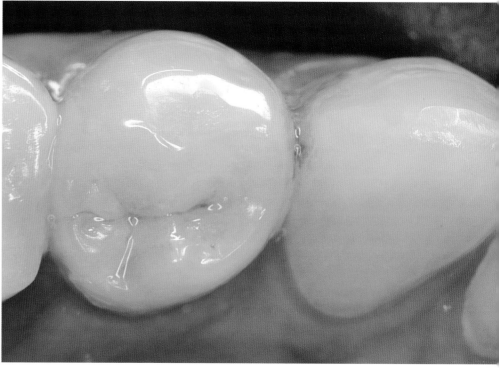

This 48-year-old patient had recurrent decay around an old amalgam filling. A porcelain inlay was selected to replace, reinforce, and support the weakened tooth structure.

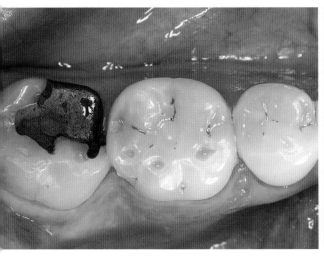 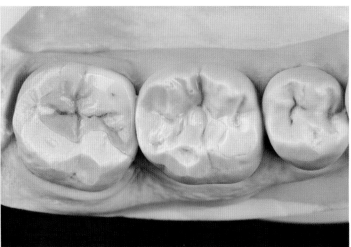 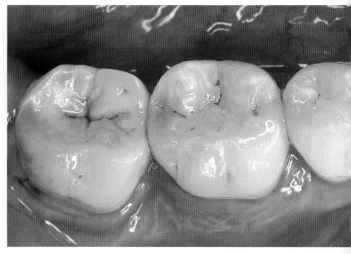

Onlays are like inlays but cover larger portions of the tooth. This custom-made filling functions as a cavity overlay and can be made of composite, porcelain, or gold. These restorations are sometimes referred to as *partial crowns* because they cover one or more cusps or the entire biting surface of the tooth. The advantages of these restorations are superior fit, improved contours, and increased durability. They are usually selected to replace and repair moderate to severe tooth decay or recurring decay on existing cracked or worn large fillings. The overlay is bonded inside and outside the cavity with adhesive cement, which can strengthen the damaged or weakened areas of the tooth. These restorations are usually prepared and fabricated in two visits to the dentist, though some dentists have computer-aided design and manufacturing systems that allow fabrication and cementation in one visit.

This patient had extensive decay around an existing cracked amalgam filling that replaced a cusp on a lower molar. A porcelain onlay was a conservative selection to fill this large cavity without having to use a crown. The divots in the cusps of the molars were restored with tooth-colored composite. An acrylic bite guard to be worn at night was also designed for his lower teeth to prevent further damage.

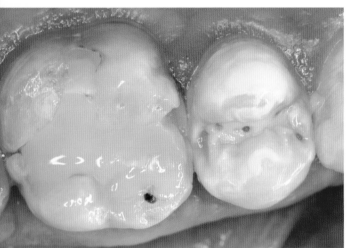 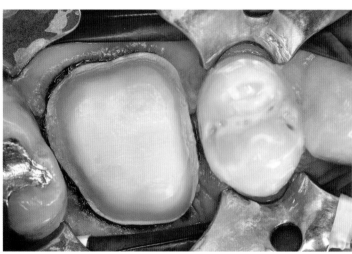 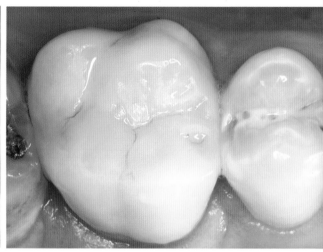

A *crown* is a tooth-shaped cover that replaces and supports a tooth that has been fractured and/or severely damaged by decay. These custom-made restorations can be made of porcelain, composite, alloy, or gold. If a large area of the tooth is missing, damaged, or decayed, a foundation called a *buildup* may be required before placing a crown. Usually the buildup is composed of a tooth-colored filling material such as composite or resin-modified glass ionomer, which gives the tooth proper dimension and body to retain the crown. Crowns are usually prepared and fabricated in two visits to the dentist, though some dentists have computer-aided design and manufacturing systems that allow fabrication and cementation in one visit.

This patient had an existing large composite filling that fractured. A composite buildup was used to provide proper dimension for the preparation. An all-ceramic crown was selected to restore the tooth to its original contour (shape) and color.

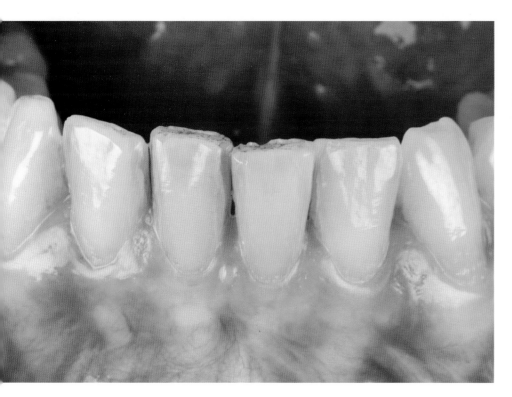
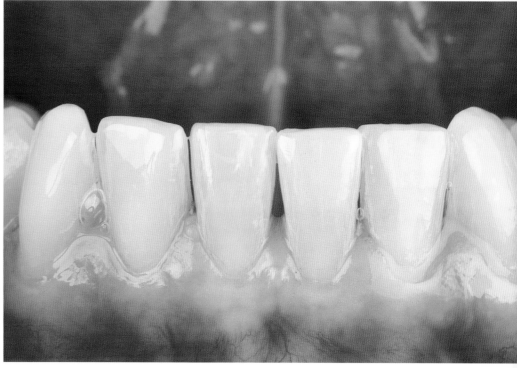

Esthetic tooth contouring is a conservative dental procedure for altering the length, size, shape, or position of misaligned front teeth. This procedure can involve removing small amounts of tooth enamel (the outer covering of the tooth) in order to eliminate small imperfections such as chips, fractures, worn edges, and shallow pits or grooves on your front teeth. Tooth contouring requires that you have normal, healthy teeth and is not appropriate for teeth with decay, root canals, or unhealthy gum tissue. Esthetic contouring can be performed with photography for more detailed analysis and may require several 1-hour visits. These minor adjustments can improve the feel, bite, alignment, and appearance of your teeth. This procedure can be used in conjunction with other esthetic procedures or after orthodontic treatment to enhance and balance your smile.

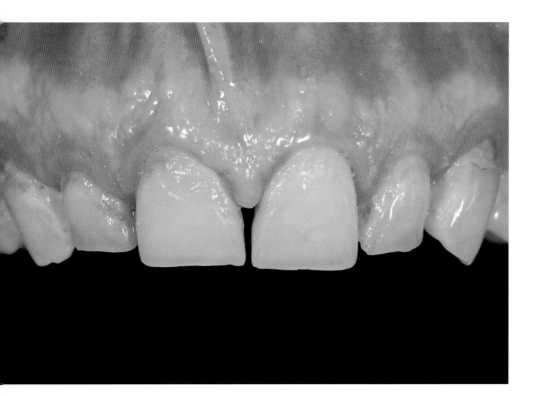 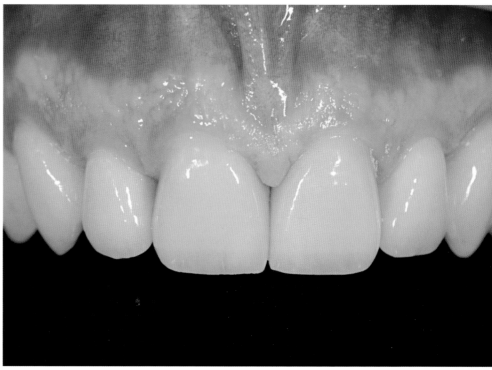

Veneers are custom-made thin shells of tooth-colored materials (composite or porcelain) that can be bonded to the front surface and sometimes back surface of your teeth to improve your smile. These shells can be used to restore teeth that are decayed, fractured, discolored, malformed, or worn. Also, they can provide esthetic solutions for closing spaces, modifying bite relationships, and altering tooth size, shape, length, alignment, color, and contour. Generally, veneers made of porcelain are more resistant to fracture than composite and do not change color or stain.

This 45-year-old woman wanted to improve her smile. Minimal preparations were performed in the enamel on her front teeth, and porcelain veneers were designed in the laboratory and bonded to her teeth at a subsequent visit.

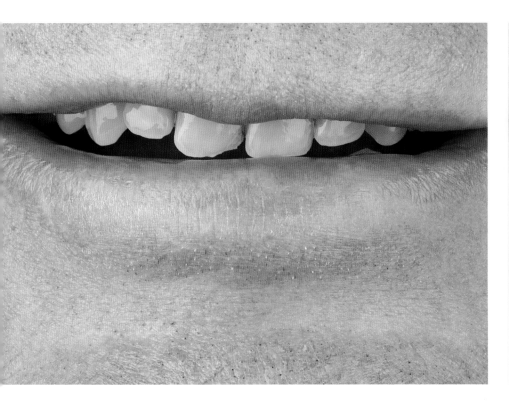 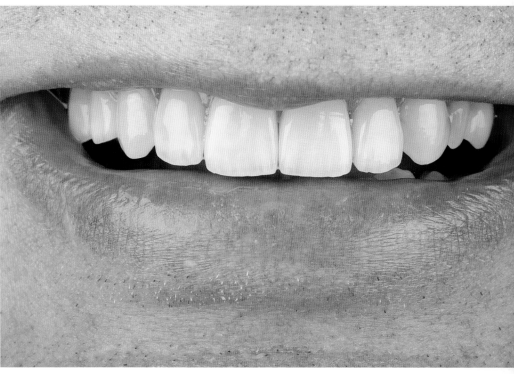

Wear and tear has a shortening and aging effect on your teeth and your smile. Attractive and younger-looking smiles have one thing in common: length. Tooth length also plays an important role in function, phonetics, and lip contour and facial esthetics.

This 54-year-old patient was concerned with his older-looking smile and appearance. His front teeth were not visible upon smiling or speaking and appeared stained, worn, and out of proportion. The patient selected a conservative treatment of bleaching and placement of four porcelain veneers on the front teeth. By increasing his smile dimensions, a younger-looking and attractive smile was achieved.

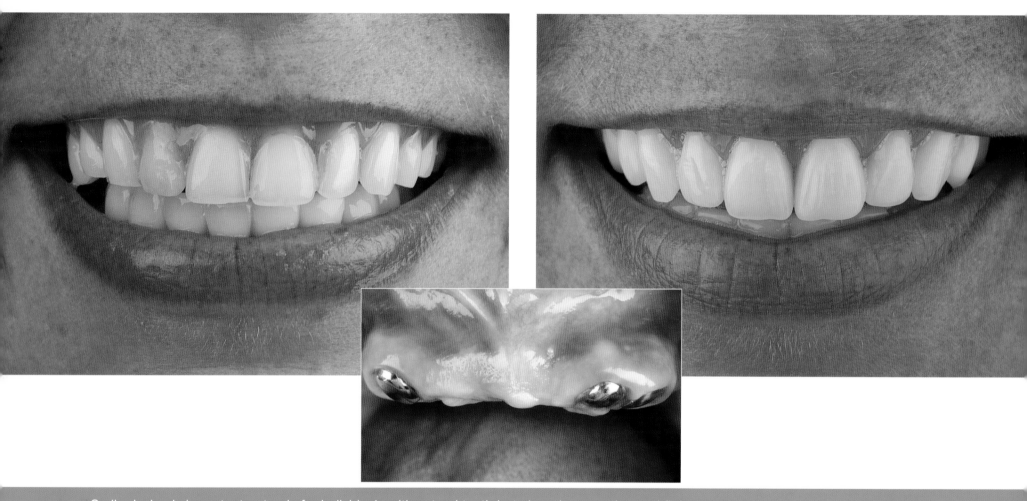

Smile design is important not only for individuals with natural teeth but also when creating and fitting an esthetic denture. *Dentures* are prosthetic dental appliances that are designed to replace missing teeth and their surrounding gums and bone. There are two main types of dentures: complete dentures and overdentures. Complete dentures replace all teeth and can be placed immediately after removal of the natural teeth or after a healing period. Overdentures are similar to complete dentures but use one or more remaining natural teeth that are cut down and used for support and retention of the denture. A modern overdenture can be designed to be implant supported. Teeth or implants underlying a denture preserve bone and improve the retention, stability, and support of the denture while improving facial support, function, and speech.

This 42-year-old woman wanted a more attractive smile and an improved bite. Her existing overdenture was unattractive and ill-fitting. An esthetic overdenture was designed for the individual size, shape, characterization, and position of her replacement teeth.

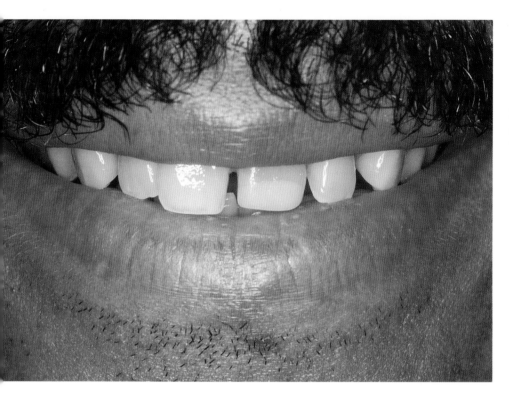
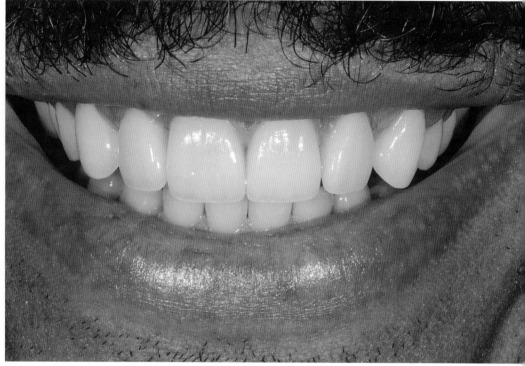

This 37-year old cardiologist was embarrassed to smile because of his gaps and misaligned teeth. Porcelain veneers were selected with only minor tooth preparation, and treatment was complete after only two appointments. This attractive smile was life changing to this professional in his career and social life.

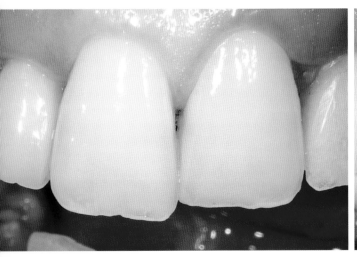 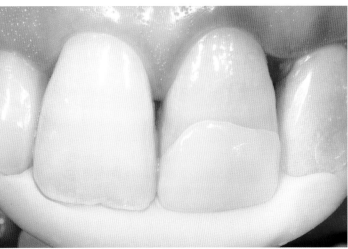 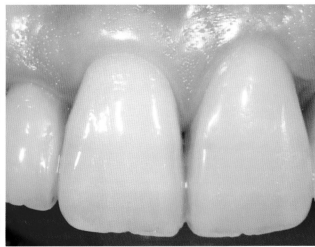

Composite veneers can be fabricated in the laboratory or formed by your dentist directly on the tooth. Laboratory-processed composite veneers have superior physical and optical qualities compared with direct composite veneers. However, direct composite veneering is sometimes a desirable option because it can be more conservative, requires less treatment time, and is more affordable. Also, direct composite veneers can be used as a transitional prototype to determine the esthetic parameters (eg, form, color, length, and contour), phonetics, and function of the restoration. This allows the patient to visualize the result and test-drive the restoration before completion with a porcelain veneer.

This 30-year-old patient was concerned about the malposition of his central incisor. Several thin layers of different tooth-colored composite resins were bonded to the unprepared tooth, improving the symmetry of his incisors.

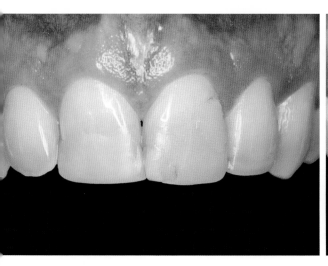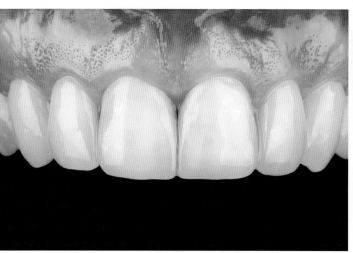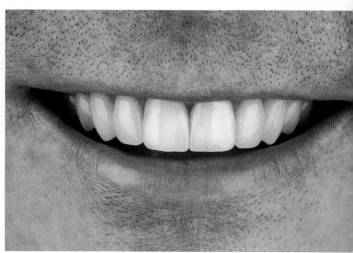

This patient wanted hand-crafted composite veneers to change the shape, color, and alignment of his natural teeth. Tooth-colored composite was directly formed and layered to create 10 composite veneers. This long-term result after 12 years is a function of expertise combined with excellent oral hygiene and routine maintenance visits by the patient.

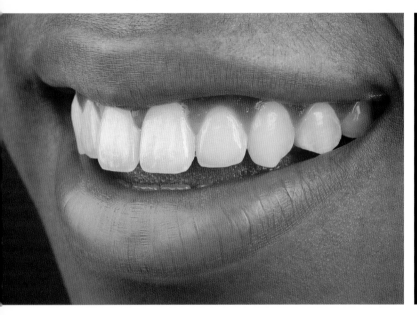
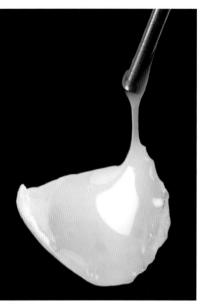
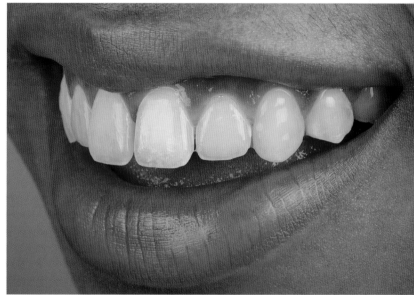

This college student was concerned about the shape and contour of her canine after having her braces removed. Without tooth preparation, a thin porcelain veneer was designed to give a natural form and contour. The veneer was bonded to the tooth with light-sensitive composite resin that was hardened using a special curing light.

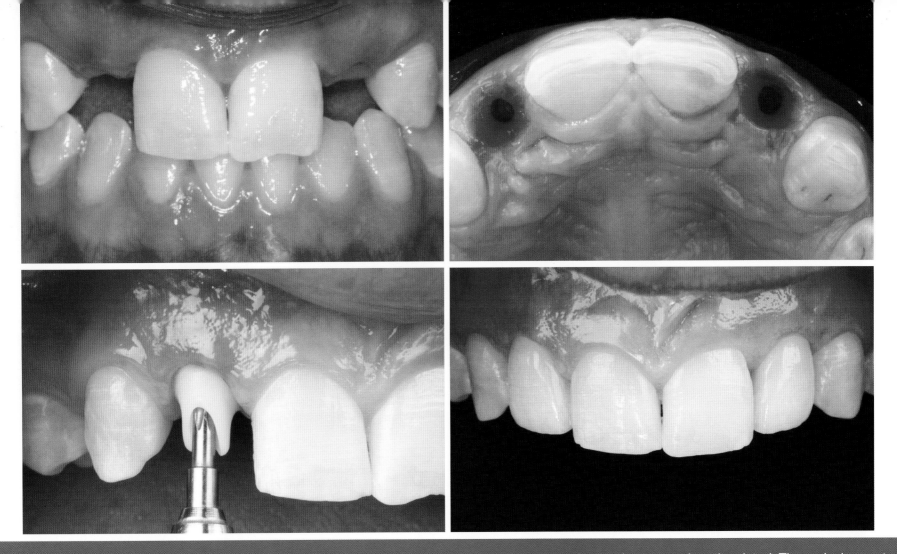

Dental implants are screw- or cylinder-like surgical devices that can be placed in the jaw where the previous natural tooth existed. These devices act as an artificial tooth root. An implant can be placed immediately after removal of a tooth or at a second surgery depending on the general health of the patient, quality and amount of supporting bone, location in the arch, bite forces from other teeth, and the preference of the surgeon and dentist. The implant and bone are allowed to bond together (osseointegrate) for 4 to 6 months to form an anchor for the artificial tooth. During this time, a temporary tooth replacement or healing cap can be worn over the implant site. After healing, an abutment is secured to the implant with a screw, and a dental crown is cemented over the abutment.

Dental implants can provide a strong foundation for a single tooth (single-tooth implant) or multiple teeth (implant-supported bridges) and can stabilize a denture (implant-supported fixed or removable dentures).

This college student had congenitally missing lateral incisors (missing from birth) and had received orthodontic treatment to align the adjacent teeth but did not want to have his adjacent teeth compromised to support fixed bridges. In a period of 6 months, the patient's confidence in his smile was restored along with normal function with single-tooth implant placements.

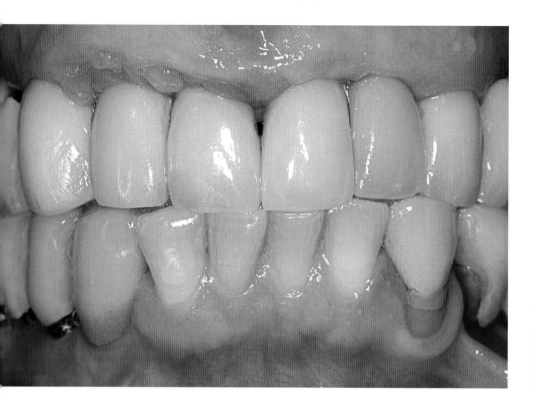
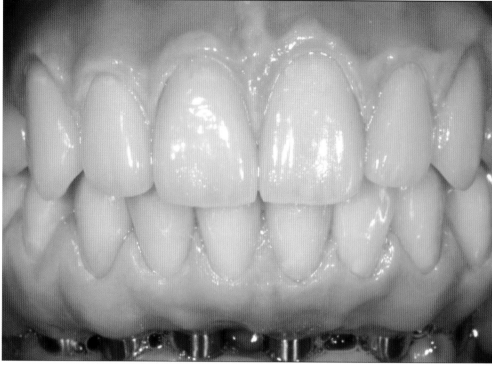

The esthetic solution for restoring an entire arch of compromised and missing teeth can be a fixed or removable overdenture. A fixed overdenture has an acrylic base with a metal substructure that is attached to four or more implants with screws. Another type of fixed overdenture uses a metal or ceramic core with porcelain on the tooth surfaces. Both are referred to as *implant-supported fixed overdentures*.

A removable overdenture has an acrylic base with adapters on its underside that engage small attachments on the implants. Another type of removable overdenture utilizes a metal bar that joins the implants and a denture with several small clips that clasp the bar. This type of overdenture can be removed by the wearer on a daily basis for oral hygiene access and is referred to as an *implant-supported removable overdenture*.

This successful businessman was concerned about the esthetics and function of his teeth after having multiple dental retreatments. Implant-supported fixed overdentures were the solution for aligning his bite and creating a life-changing improvement in his smile.

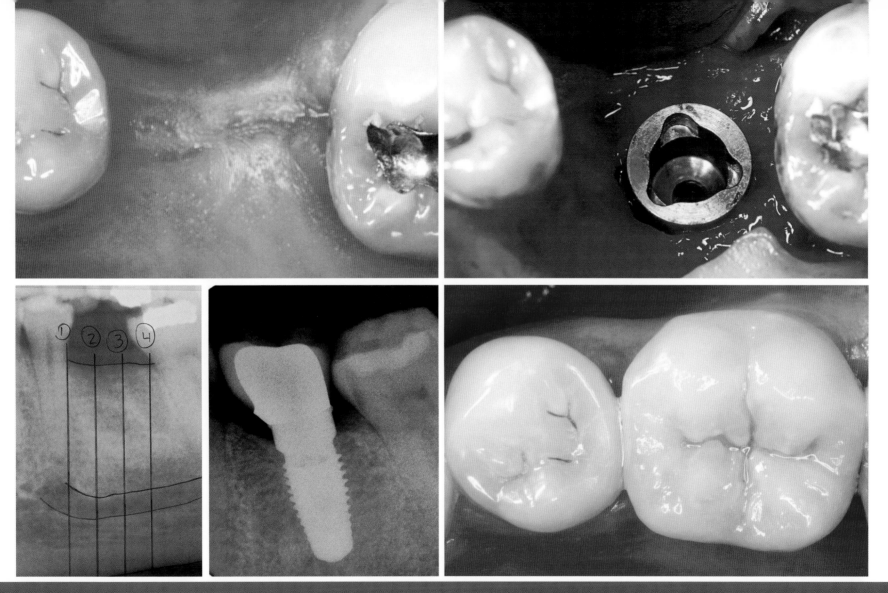

This 40-year-old patient was concerned about a missing lower molar. The tooth had been removed 1 year before, and he noticed that the upper molar was moving down into the empty space. His previous dentist suggested that a three-unit bridge would be the best option for treatment and that his insurance would cover most of the cost. However, he was not interested in having the adjacent teeth cut down for support of a bridge. After researching the Internet for potential treatment options, he decided to get another opinion. A preliminary x-ray was taken to determine the quality and quantity of the bone, the location of vital anatomical structures, and the position of the roots of adjacent teeth. After a complete evaluation, an implant-supported crown was selected for treatment. A computed tomography (CT) scan, a 3D x-ray, was used to determine the most precise position of the implant. This x-ray scanning device provides images by section, allowing for the best placement position for the implant. After 7 years of good function (see 7-year postoperative x-ray, bottom center), he was glad he chose the least invasive option for his treatment.

37

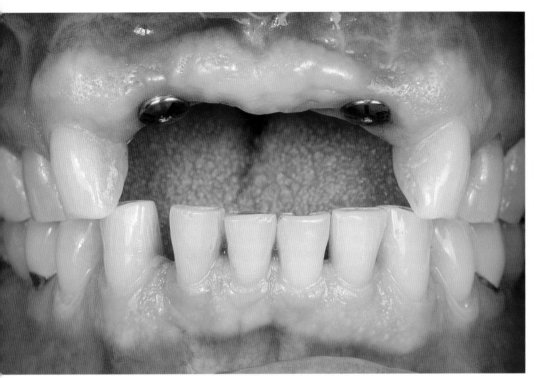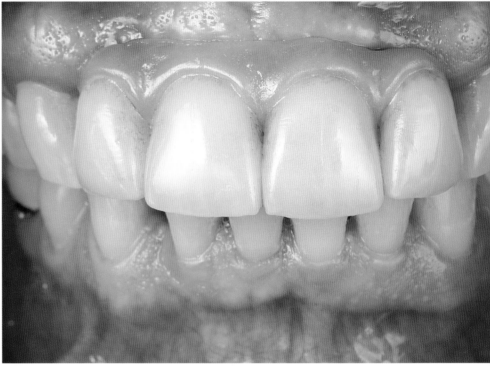

This 65-year-old man lost his front teeth from a failed dental bridge. He had always been concerned about the unesthetic appearance of the bridge when he smiled. An implant-supported fixed bridge (screw-retained) was selected to restore the space. This fixed bridge was composed of ceramic teeth and a base with a metal substructure that was attached to two implants with screws. The patient was elated to finally have optimal function and the smile he had always wanted.

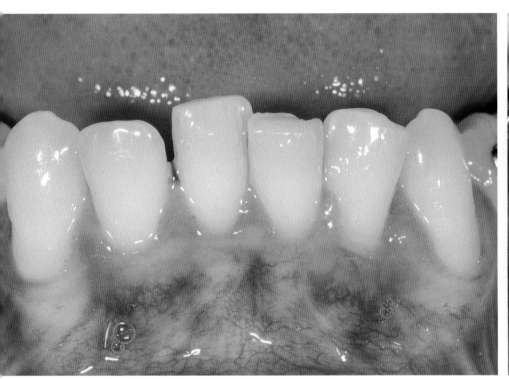
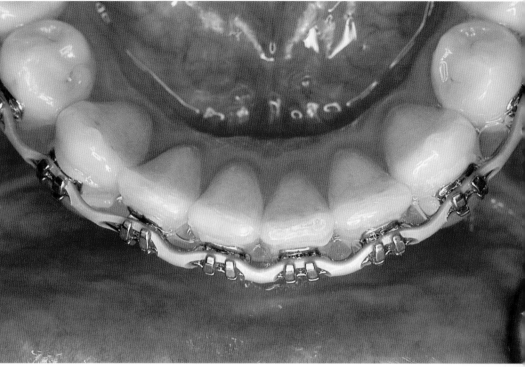

Teeth can shift with age, and many adult patients have difficulty properly cleaning their teeth. Misaligned teeth increase the chances of food, plaque, and calculus buildup and predispose the individual to periodontal disease and jaw pain. Instead of overaggressive tooth reduction to align teeth with cosmetic restorations, today's informed adult sees braces as a worthwhile investment of time in exchange for decades of uncompromised straight teeth.

This 36-year-old woman was concerned about her crowded and uneven lower teeth. It took less than 2 years to align her teeth and bite and give her a more attractive smile.

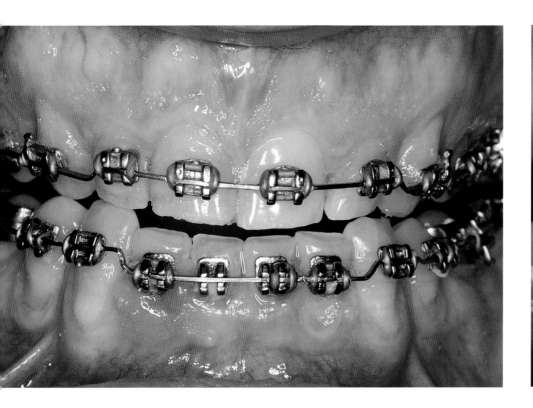 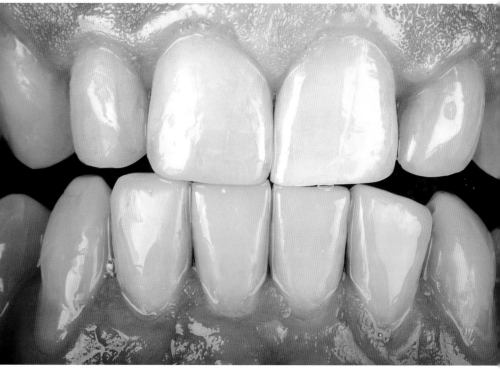

Age should not be a consideration for orthodontic treatment because a healthy bite is as important at age 50 years as it is at age 15 years. There are a variety of orthodontic appliances available, including metal braces, tooth-colored braces, braces that are positioned behind the teeth, clear aligners, and other devices. Orthodontic treatment not only aligns crowded teeth but can also resolve malocclusion (bad bite), speech difficulties, periodontal conditions, facial imbalance or asymmetry, grinding or clenching of teeth (bruxism), and chewing disorders (eg, temporomandibular disorders). However, orthodontics for adults may require additional time and more than one dental professional to resolve complex conditions.

This 52-year-old patient was concerned about the alignment of his teeth and his bite. A combination of orthodontic treatment and veneers corrected his bite while improving his appearance and self-confidence.

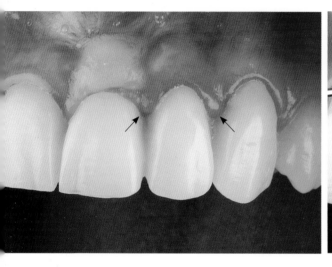 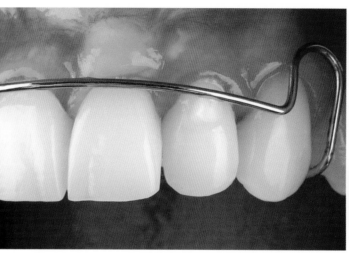 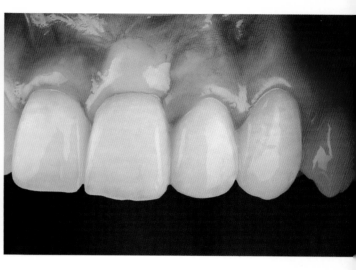

The gum levels of teeth not only determine the esthetic potential for the smile but also define the crown length available for a restoration. Gum line asymmetries are often treated surgically (periodontal crown lengthening or orthognathic surgery), but orthodontic treatment can also be an effective method of leveling the gum line architecture before restoring the teeth. *Forced eruption* is an orthodontic procedure of raising the root with gentle continuous force. Localized gum line asymmetries can sometimes be treated with this technique. An isolated tooth can be used to raise the gums and bone around the tooth, correcting gum defects. The part of the gum that fills the space between teeth is called the *interdental papilla*.

This 41-year-old woman had a deficient papilla between her incisors *(arrows)*, making the gum level and contours unnatural looking. By using forced eruption, the papilla length and shape were modified. After 3 months, the gum contours were dramatically improved and ready for definitive restorations.

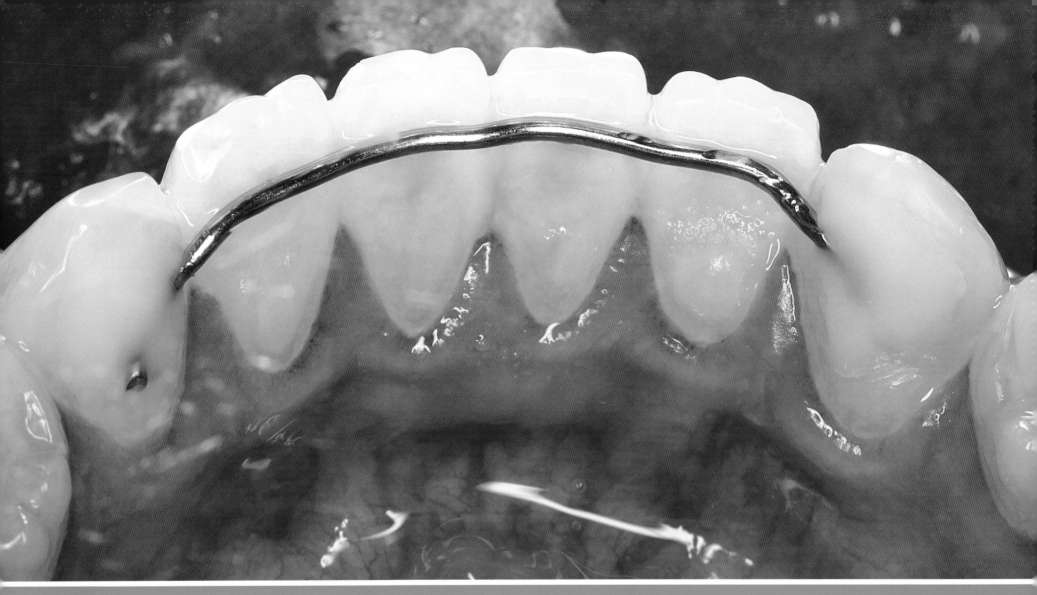

After orthodontic treatment is completed and the braces are removed, a fixed orthodontic wire is often bonded to the teeth to ensure that the position and spacing of the teeth remain the same. Improper care can result in infected gums. A floss threader can be used to insert and maneuver the floss and clean the surfaces between the teeth. If plaque continues to build up, it can become mineralized to form calculus deposits (tartar) around the retainer wire and the teeth and cause periodontal disease.

This 25-year-old patient was negligent in routine brushing and flossing around his retainer, resulting in gingivitis and bad breath.

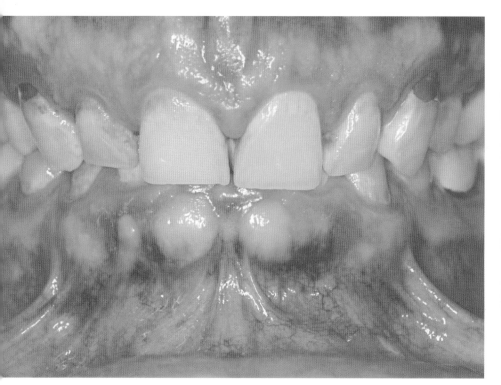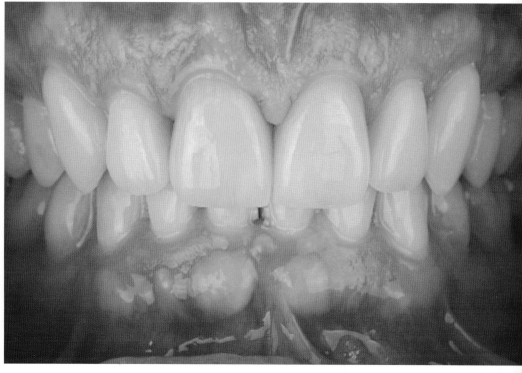

Some patients seek only a more attractive smile, while others want reliable teeth that allow them to chew and eat comfortably. A complete dental rehabilitation or full-mouth reconstruction involves restoring, replacing, or rebuilding all of the remaining teeth in the upper and lower jaws and properly aligning the jaws. Oral conditions that may require rehabilitation include worn, chipped, or broken teeth, failing dental restorations, widespread tooth decay, significant tooth wear caused by grinding or corrosive components (eg, gastric reflux, bulimia), and a chewing system that has declined. This series of procedures, known as *reconstruction*, involves restoring the function of your teeth, jaws, and muscles as a whole. Treatment may require the use of crowns, bridges, veneers, partial dentures, or complete dentures on natural teeth and/or dental implants.

This middle-aged executive had severe wear and attrition on all of his teeth and desired an improved bite and more attractive smile. After restoration of all of his natural teeth with all-ceramic crowns to improve their dimensions, color, and contours, the patient was extremely pleased with his balanced bite and beautiful smile.

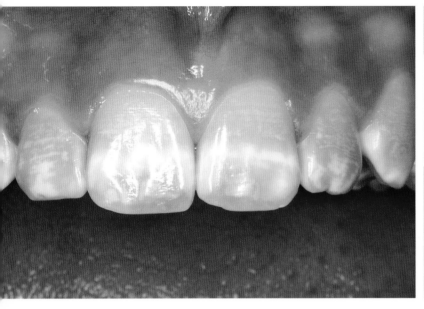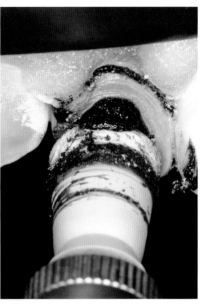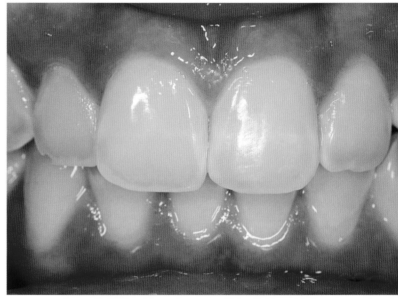

Alterations in tooth color can have a variety of causes including superficial and internal staining. Cosmetic treatments of these color alterations range from conservative to more invasive procedures. Conservative treatments include chemical treatments (bleaching) and chemical and micromechanical abrasive treatments (including enamel microabrasion), while invasive treatments include composite or porcelain veneers and porcelain crowns. Treatment considerations should begin with the most conservative and progress as needed to more invasive alternatives depending on the depth of the staining.

This 26-year-old patient had a condition called *fluorosis*. This condition occurs with the intake of excessive concentrations of fluoride during formation of the crown, leaving a white speckled mottling appearance on the tooth. A procedure known as *enamel microabrasion* was selected for eliminating the discolorations. This process involves using several applications of an acidic substance in combination with an abrasive agent. The patient was very pleased with the results and now smiles with confidence.

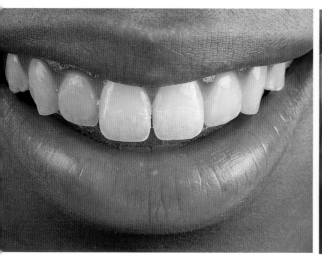
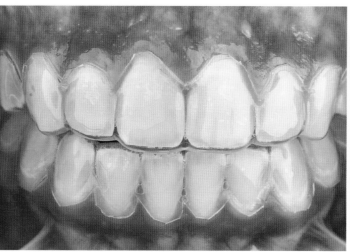
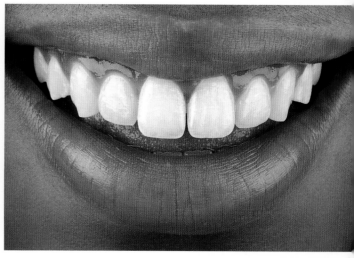

Dental bleaching, also known as *tooth whitening*, is a chemical process of applying oxidizing agents to the tooth surface that penetrate the enamel and dentin and break down stain deposits, resulting in alterations in the tooth color. There are many methods for bleaching teeth, including in-office bleaching, at-home bleaching, and over-the-counter remedies. Before initiating any bleaching procedure, you should have your dentist take a thorough dental history and evaluate your teeth and gums. Bleaching is most effective for yellow discolored teeth and is not recommended if teeth have decay or the gums are infected. Also, because bleaching is not effective on tooth-colored restorations, any fillings you have may require replacement to match the new brighter shade. Bleaching may require periodic touch-up applications.

This college student was unhappy about the staining on her healthy teeth after the removal of her braces. Professional at-home bleaching was performed using custom bleaching trays and a 10% carbamide peroxide gel. The yellow stains were removed, unveiling a beautiful and healthy smile.

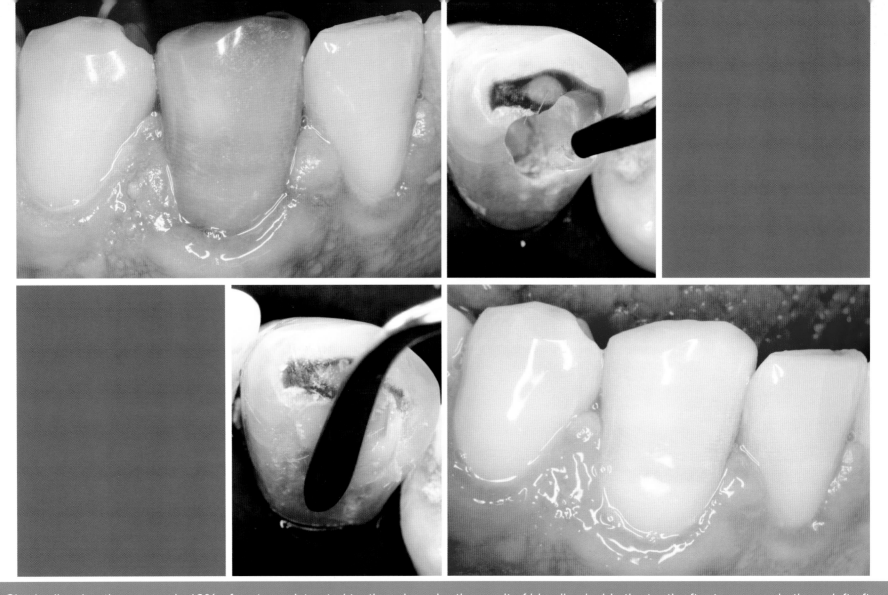

Shade discoloration occurs in 10% of root canal–treated teeth and can be the result of bleeding inside the tooth after trauma, pulp tissue left after treatment, drugs used in the root canal treatment, and staining from dental cements or materials. Nonvital bleaching is a procedure for treating discolored root canal–treated teeth and involves an in-office procedure or the "walking bleach technique" or a combination of both. The treatment consists of placing a high concentration of bleaching solution or gel inside a tooth and usually requires several applications.

The "walking bleach technique" was selected for this 65-year-old patient. After the root canal was sealed with a glass-ionomer intermediate filling material, a 35% hydrogen peroxide gel was placed into the nerve chamber and sealed with a temporary filling. After three visits, the discolorations were eliminated, and the patient was elated with the color match to his adjacent teeth.

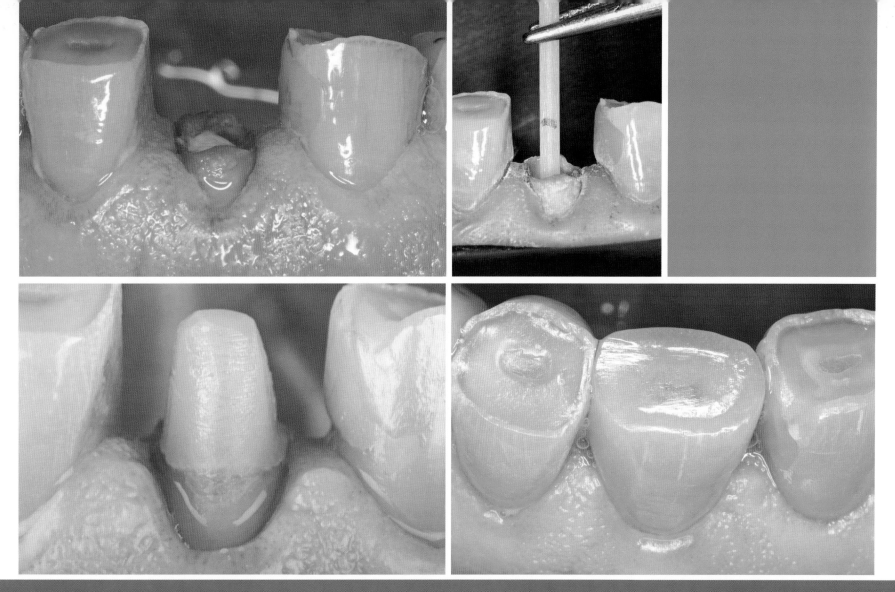

A *post and core* is a type of dental restoration that is used when there is inadequate tooth structure remaining to support a traditional restoration. These restorations can be used to replace the missing portion of severely broken-down teeth due to fracture or decay and require the tooth to be treated with root canal therapy. Posts come in a variety of shapes, sizes, and materials. Traditionally, posts have been fabricated using different metals; however, current evidence indicates the use of fiber-reinforced resin post systems for improved clinical success. The composite post is inserted and bonded into a prepared channel in the root and is used to anchor a composite core. Placing a composite post and core strengthens the tooth and provides better retention and support for the crown.

This 72-year-old patient fractured his root canal–treated tooth, which was restored in one appointment with a composite post and core. An all-ceramic crown was placed at a subsequent visit.

Definitions of Recognized Dental Specialties*

Dental public health The science and art of preventing and controlling dental diseases and promoting dental health through organized community efforts. This form of dental practice serves the *community* as a patient rather than the individual. It is concerned with the dental health education of the public, with applied dental research, and with the administration of group dental care programs as well as the prevention and control of dental diseases on a community basis.

Endodontics The branch of dentistry concerned with the morphology, physiology, and pathology of the human dental pulp and periradicular tissues. Its study and practice encompass the basic and clinical sciences, including biology of the normal pulp; the etiology, diagnosis, prevention, and treatment of diseases; and injuries of the pulp and associated periradicular conditions.

Oral and maxillofacial pathology The specialty of dentistry and discipline of pathology that deals with the nature, identification, and management of diseases affecting the oral and maxillofacial regions. It is a science that investigates the causes, processes, and effects of these diseases. The practice of oral pathology includes research and diagnosis of diseases using clinical, radiographic, microscopic, biochemical, or other examinations.

Oral and maxillofacial radiology The specialty of dentistry and discipline of radiology concerned with the production and interpretation of images and data produced by all modalities of radiant energy that are used for the diagnosis and management of diseases, disorders, and conditions of the oral and maxillofacial region.

Oral and maxillofacial surgery The specialty of dentistry that includes the diagnosis and surgical and adjunctive treatment of diseases, injuries, and defects involving both the functional and esthetic aspects of the hard and soft tissues of the oral and maxillofacial region.

Orthodontics and dentofacial orthopedics The dental specialty that includes the diagnosis, prevention, interception, and correction of malocclusion as well as neuromuscular and skeletal abnormalities of the developing or mature orofacial structures.

Pediatric dentistry An age-defined specialty that provides both primary and comprehensive preventive and therapeutic oral health care for infants and children through adolescence, including those with special health care needs.

Periodontics The specialty of dentistry that encompasses the prevention, diagnosis, and treatment of diseases of the supporting and surrounding tissues of the teeth or their substitutes and the maintenance of the health, function, and esthetics of these structures and tissues.

Prosthodontics The dental specialty pertaining to the diagnosis, treatment planning, rehabilitation, and maintenance of the oral function, comfort, appearance, and health of patients with clinical conditions associated with missing or deficient teeth and/or oral and maxillofacial tissues using biocompatible substitutes.

*Approved by the Council on Dental Education and Licensure, American Dental Association.

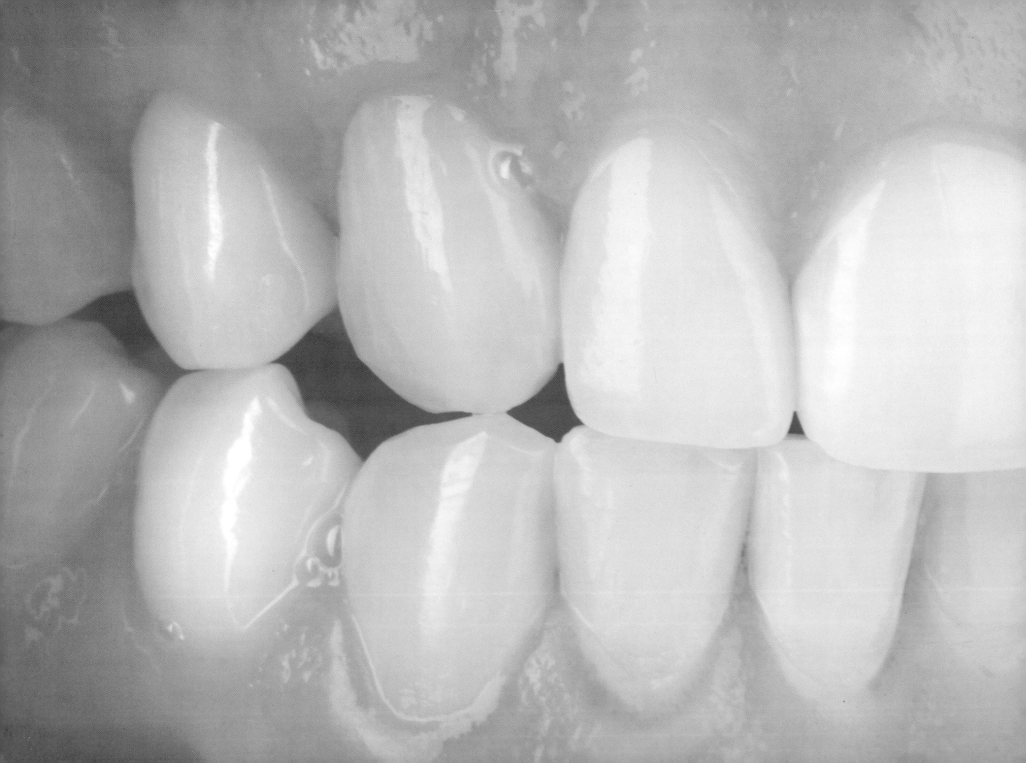